# Germ Smart

## Children's Activities in Disease Prevention

**Judith K. Scheer, EdS, CHES**

*Illustrated by Nina Paley*

ETR Associates
Santa Cruz, California
1990

## About ETR Associates

ETR Associates (Education, Training and Research) is a nonprofit organization committed to fostering the health, well-being and cultural diversity of individuals, families, schools and communities. The publishing program of ETR Associates provides books and materials that empower young people and adults with the skills to make positive health choices. We invite health professionals to learn more about our high-quality publishing, training and research programs by contacting us at P.O. Box 1830, Santa Cruz, CA 95061-1830.

## About the Author

Judith K. Scheer, EdS, CHES, has been a health teacher at the elementary and high school levels and a university professor and supervisor of student teachers. She has been a teacher, curriculum writer and trainer for Growing Healthy, as well as a Quest trainer in the Skills for Living program. Ms. Scheer is also the author of *You and Me Tobacco Free: Children's Activities in Tobacco Awareness* and *Into Adolescence: Living Without Tobacco* (ETR Associates, 1990).

## About the Activity Series

This is just one of many titles in the creative **Children's Activity Series** from ETR Associates. Each fun-filled activity book has a companion poster, available in bulk quantities, to reinforce its important health message. Color them in! Hang them up! Send them home! These resource books and posters are designed to help you build students' health skills in school *and* at home! For more information and a free catalog, call toll-free 1-800-321-4407.

10   9   8   7   6   5   4

Cover Design: Julia Chiapella

Title No. 586

**Library of Congress Cataloging-in-Publication Data**

Scheer, Judith K.
    Germ smart : children's activities in disease prevention /
Judith K. Scheer ; illustrated by Nina Paley.
        p. cm.
    ISBN 1-56071-015-2
    1. Health Education (Preschool)—United States. 2. Health
Education (Elementary)—United States. 3. Early childhood
education—Activity programs. 4. Germ theory of disease.
I. Paley, Nina. II. Title
LB1140.5.H4S34      1990
372. 3'7—dc20                                    90-6295

# Contents

# Series Introduction

The **Children's Activity Series** promotes awareness about health, family life and cultural diversity for children in kindergarten through third grade. Each book focuses on a topic that can be difficult for elementary school teachers to address. Activities have been specifically designed to help children grow into adults who:

- feel good about themselves;

- interact with others;

- choose a healthful lifestyle;

- avoid tobacco, alcohol and other drugs;

- are open to the diversity of our world and its cultures; and

- contribute in a responsible way to society.

The books in this series are written to enhance an established curriculum, rather than to serve as the curriculum. They offer ideas for hands-on activities for teachers to integrate into the primary-level curriculum. Teachers can use the various interactive and lively activities as-is or adapt them to meet the needs of their specific situations.

The format of each activity is designed to help teachers easily prepare for the busy hands-on work. The **Get Ready, Get Set...** section outlines any advance preparation needed to conduct the activity. All items for student use are clearly identified in the **Materials for Children** section. The steps for the process of the activity are detailed in the **Here We Go!** section. Reproducible masters for student activity sheets and teacher patterns are found at the end of the activity.

The books in the **Children's Activity Series** are developed by authors familiar with both the content and process appropriate for primary school students in specific topic areas. And most importantly, the activities have been tested with children and have proven to be both educational and FUN.

# Author's Introduction

What can be more exciting than providing children with the skills needed to begin taking responsibility for their own health? This foundation will certainly affect the quality of each day of their lives.

The purpose of this book is to provide you with ideas for helping children learn what germs are, how the body fights disease and infections and how our behaviors can interrupt or enhance the body's natural ability to fight intruders.

We begin with an activity that builds awareness of vulnerability to disease—a bulletin board that is sure to attract outside interest, as well. A building activity introduces the concept of cells and demonstrations. Experiments address what germs are, how they are spread and how they create damage.

To provide children with a sense of control over vulnerability to illness, activities that teach the basics of controlling the spread of germs are provided. Children learn to cover coughs and sneezes, wash hands properly and

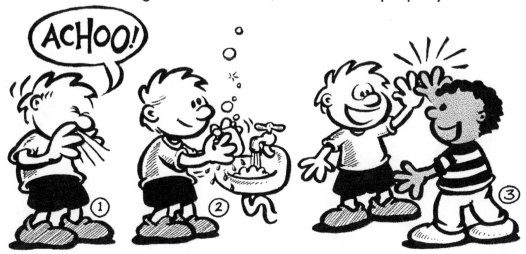

care for the skin. They are taught to avoid high-risk situations such as blood-mixing games.

Through roleplay and puppetry, the immune system is introduced. By understanding basic concepts about the function of the immune system, children begin to respect the body as a "miracle machine." This attitude motivates children to care for the machine by making wise health choices. A health continuum underscores how personal decisions affect health on a day-to-day basis.

I encourage you to present these activities with lots of additional attention to building self-esteem. Include time to listen to each child's perceptions and experiences, recognizing that different cultures and families have their own beliefs and health practices.

The body is a wonderful machine. Knowledge of how it works and skill in keeping it at peak efficiency give our children confidence, security and freedom to become all that they can be.

*Judy Scheer*

# 1 Germs Cause Disease

## Purpose

To help children understand that disease is a part of life and is experienced by everyone.

## In a Nutshell

Children crumple pieces of paper to represent their experience of disease. They use the paper to create a bulletin board display.

## Get Ready, Get Set...

• Gather needed materials: felt marker, 4-foot piece of butcher paper or newsprint.
• Draw a life-size outline of a child's body on butcher paper and post it in the front of the room.
• Title a large bulletin board **Germ Victories!**
• Prepare word cards using *New Words*.
• Gather materials for children.

## Materials for Children

★ 6 in. x 8 in. pieces of scrap paper or newspaper, 10 per child
★ stapler, tacks or tape

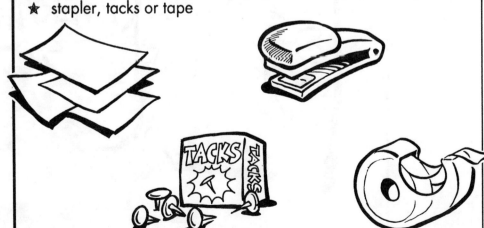

# Here We Go!

1. Begin with all children standing. Ask if there are any children in the class who have *never* been sick. Have those children sit down. Ask children if they know anyone in their families who has *never* been sick. Tell children who have a family member who has never been sick to sit down.

   How many children are still standing? Ask children who would like to always be healthy to sit down. Do children think it's important to stay healthy?

   Tell children to think about the reasons people stay healthy and don't get sick. Are people who are usually healthy just lucky? Are there things people can do to help themselves stay well? Encourage children to share their ideas about how to stay well.

2. Ask children to name some of the sicknesses they know. Guide them to include common communicable and noncommunicable diseases such as *mumps, chicken pox, colds, flu, polio, cancer, measles, diabetes.*

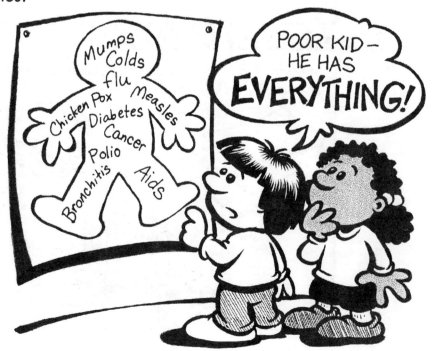

As each disease is named, write its name in large print on the life-size body outline.

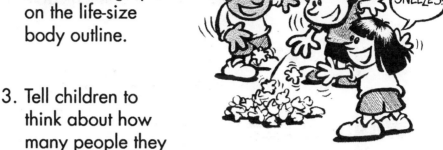

3. Tell children to think about how many people they know who have had each disease. Pass out at least 10 pieces of scrap paper to each child.

Tell children to crumple up a piece of paper for each person they think of (no names, please!) and put it in a pile on the floor. The pile will get bigger as each disease is named.

4. Tell children that when someone gets sick, germs have won a battle in that person's body. Have groups of children attach the crumpled papers to the bulletin board.

Explain that each crumpled piece of paper stands for a germ victory. Label the bulletin board **Germ Victories**.

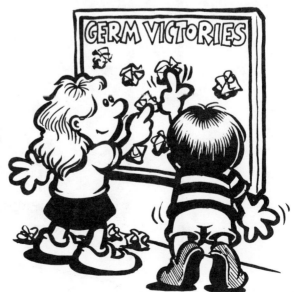

5. Tell children that germs can make anyone sick, but there are things we can do that will help us win the battle against germs. Tell children they are going to learn ways to fight

germs and reduce germ victories.

Save the child's body outline for use in teaching about communicable and noncommunicable diseases.

## New Words

disease, germ, healthy, sick, sickness, victory

## Where It Fits

health, science

# 2 Two Kinds of Germs

## Purpose

To help children conceptualize how viruses destroy cells.

## In a Nutshell

Children work in groups to build a structure out of cells. Then they examine orange segments to identify cells. A demonstration shows how viruses destroy cells.

## Get Ready, Get Set...

• Gather needed materials: several 3-4-inch toothpicks, 15 building blocks per group, large plastic egg (L'eggs eggs work great!), mini-marshmallows, tennis ball.
• Place 15 mini-marshmallows inside the plastic egg. Have an additional mini-marshmallow ready to insert during demonstration.
• Prepare word cards using *New Words*.
• Gather materials for children.

## Materials for Children

★ building blocks
★ an orange segment for each child

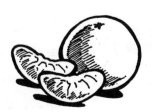
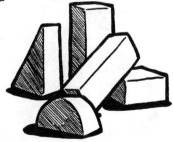

# Here We Go!

1. Tell children that bacteria are one type (or family) of germs. Most bacteria are *not* harmful. Some bacteria even help us digest our food. But some bacteria can make people very sick.

   Tell children that the name *bacteria* comes from a Greek word (*bakterion*) that means a small rod or stick. Explain that under a microscope, bacteria look like tiny sticks. Show the toothpicks to represent bacteria.

2. Tell children that viruses are another type of germ. Viruses cause some of the diseases the children may have had, such as flu and colds. They also cause measles, chicken pox, mumps and AIDS.

   Explain that viruses only grow (reproduce) when they are inside a living cell. When a lot of viruses are living inside the body, the body becomes feverish (warm) to try to destroy the viruses. If we have lots of viruses inside our bodies, we feel sick.

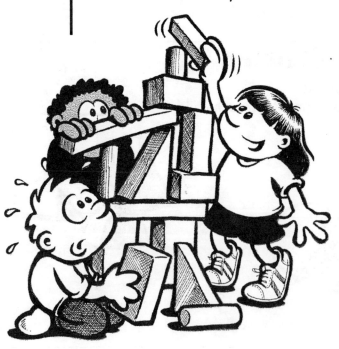

3. Divide class into groups of 4 or 5. Give each group about 15 building blocks. Tell children to think of the blocks as cells. Tell them to build something with their cells.

   Give each child an orange segment. Tell children to study the segment. If they look closely, they should be able to identify the cells of the orange. Together, these cells make a segment, and the segments make an orange.

Explain that there are different kinds of cells. All living things are made of some kind of cells.

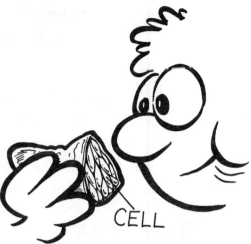

CELL

4. Show children a large plastic egg to represent a cell and a mini-marshmallow to represent a virus. Show the children how viruses destroy cells. The egg should be half-full of mini-marshmallows. Open the egg to slip the additional "virus" inside (keeping the other marshmallows carefully concealed!).

Explain that although the cell looks the same from the outside, it has been taken over by the virus. It is now a "virus factory." Soon the cell will be full of viruses.

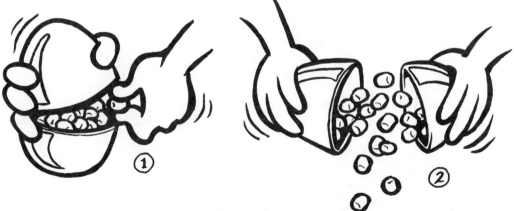

Then it will *burst* open and scatter the new viruses. As you say *burst*, pull the egg apart, allowing marshmallows to fly out.

Hold the two halves of the cell. Show children how the cell has been destroyed. What will happen to the cell that burst? (It dies.) What will the new viruses do? (find other cells to invade)

5. Show children a tennis ball to represent the size of bacteria. Compare the tennis ball to the mini-marsh-mallows that represent viruses. Point out how much bigger the bacteria are.

## New Words

bacteria, cell, fever, virus

## Where It Fits

health, science

# 3 Where Germs Hide

## Purpose

To help children recognize that germs are found almost anywhere.

## In a Nutshell

Children discuss where germs live. Samples from children's hands and mouths are collected to make germ cultures. Children draw pictures of germs and places germs hide.

## Get Ready, Get Set...

• Prepare agar plates for a germ culture. Plan to store the agar plates in a warm, dark place for several days. Prepare **Where Germs Hide** title for art display.
• Write each child's name on a small strip of paper.
• Prepare word cards using *New Words*.
• Gather materials for children.

## Materials for Children

★ cotton-tipped stick for each child
★ straight pin for each child

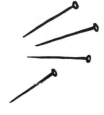

# Here We Go!

1. Tell children that some germs live outside the body. Other germs can only live inside our bodies. Ask children where outside germs might be found. (Outside germs can be found in air, water, food—on most things.)

   Ask children how these germs from outside get into our bodies to make us sick. (They can enter through body openings, such as the mouth, eyes or nose. They can also enter through breaks in our skin due to cuts, scrapes and punctures, and even dry, chapped skin that has cracked.)

   How could the inside germs from another person get into our bodies? (from mother at birth, from someone else's blood) Ask children which germs are easier to catch—inside or outside (outside).

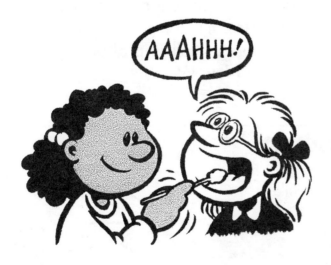

2. Explain to children that germs can grow in many places. Tell them, "We are going to grow some germs." Create a germ culture on agar plates. Collect samples from the hands or mouths of each child. Use a cotton-tipped stick to collect the germs. Use a clean one each time.

   Spread the sample on the agar. Identify the sample with a pin and the child's name. Keep cultures in a dark, warm place for several days. Discuss the appearance of the culture.

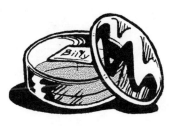

3.   Ask children what illnesses or diseases they are most afraid of. Why? Discuss their fears and ways to deal with fear. Tell children that it's important to talk to a trusted grown-up at home or at school about their fears and questions. Explain that we know how to prevent or cure many, many illnesses and diseases caused by germs.

4. Have children draw pictures of places and things where germs hide. Tell them to draw the germs, too. Post these pictures around the room, with the title **Where Germs Hide.**

## New Words

fear, inside germs, outside germs

## Where It Fits

art, health, science

# 4 | Outside Germs

## Purpose

To help children realize that outside germs are easily spread from person to person.

## In a Nutshell

Glitter is sprinkled in children's hands during a demonstration about how germs spread. Children participate in a hand-washing experiment.

## Get Ready, Get Set...

• Gather needed materials: spray bottle filled with dark colored water.
• Have soap and warm water available.
• Make a poster from the teacher page **How Germs Are Spread.**
• Prepare word cards using *New Words*.
• Gather materials for children.

### Materials for Children

★ glitter
★ white paper
★ petroleum jelly or shortening
★ ground nutmeg
★ light-colored paper towels
★ pens, pencils or crayons

## Here We Go!

1.  Sprinkle glitter on the hands of every child. (Caution children not to rub the glitter into their eyes.) Allow children to continue their usual routines for about 15 minutes.

    Have children look to see where their hands carried the glitter around the room. Tell them this is one way germs are spread. Discuss some of the other ways germs are spread (cough, sneeze, water, food, animals, insects, etc.).

2.  Illustrate what happens when people sneeze or cough. Tell children that tiny droplets are spread into the air.

    Give each child a piece of white paper. Use a spray bottle to spray colored water onto each child's paper. Have children draw a circle around the spray area.

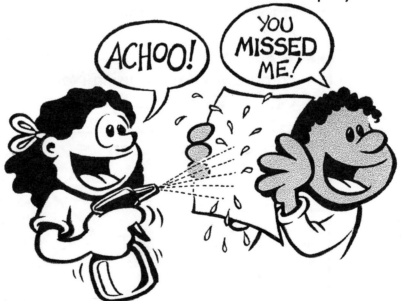

    Use the poster **How Germs Are Spread** to explain that coughing and sneezing are two ways the body gets germs out of it. But coughing and sneezing can spread germs to others. Tell children this is why it is so important to cover coughs and sneezes so the germs can't spread.

3. Tell children that germs can cause stomach problems. Germs can spread from one person to another person when we touch hands. Then when your hand touches your mouth, the germs get inside your body. If you do not wash your hands after using the bathroom, you might have germs on your hands.

You leave the germs on things you touch, just like you spread the glitter. When another person comes by and touches what you've touched, they get the germs on their skin. Review ways germs can get from the skin to inside the body (Concept 3).

4. Conduct a hand-washing experiment. Use petroleum jelly or shortening to represent skin oils. Have each child rub a 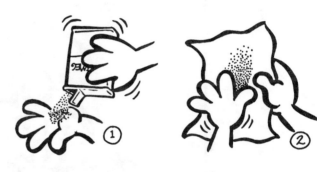 small amount on his or her hands. Sprinkle nutmeg on the children's hands. Tell children the nutmeg represents dirt and germs.

Have half the children wash their hands with cool water and no soap. Then have them dry their hands on light-colored paper towels. The nutmeg will be clearly visible on the towels. Point out to children that the cool water did not remove the dirt and germs.

Have the remaining children wash their hands with warm water and soap. Tell them to wash both sides of their hands and their fingernails. Have them rinse with warm water, then dry their hands on the light-colored paper towels. Examine the towels for signs of nutmeg. There should be none.

Lead children to conclude that washing carefully with soap and warm water removes dirt and germs trapped in the skin oils. Skin oils that are removed by washing are quickly replaced by the body.

Have the first group of children use warm water and soap to wash their hands again. They should not find any "germs" on the paper towels this time.

## New Words

cough, sneeze, stomach, touch

## Where It Fits

health, science

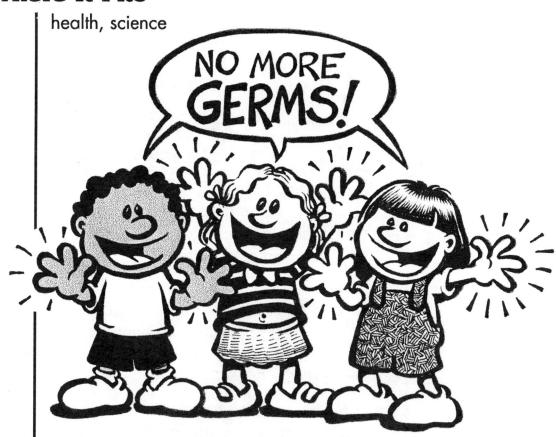

# How Germs Are Spread

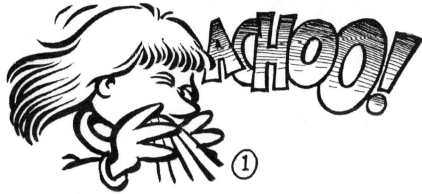

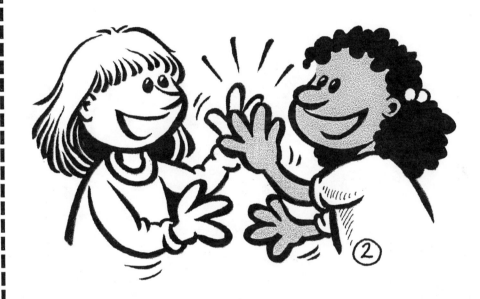

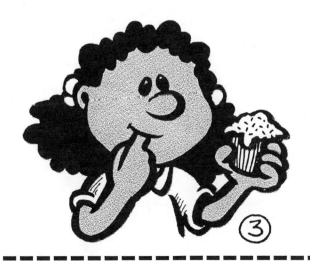

# **5** **Inside Germs**

## Purpose

To help children realize that certain kinds of germs are not easily spread from person to person.

## In a Nutshell

Children identify some common liquids. They compare these liquids to body fluids that can transmit germs.

## Get Ready, Get Set...

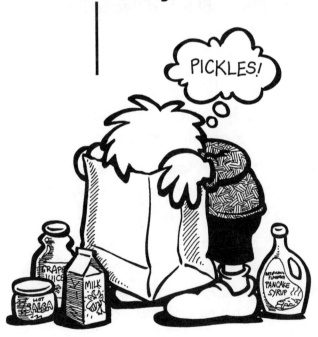

• Obtain a rubber fish or make a poster using the **Fish** teacher page.
• Fill a grocery bag with 5-6 samples or empty containers of liquids that are found in refrigerators (milk, apple juice, pickle juice, salsa, syrup.)
• Prepare word cards using *New Words*. (Select age-appropriate terms for your class.)

## Here We Go!

1. Show children the rubber fish or the **Fish** poster. Ask what happens to real fish when they are removed from water (die).

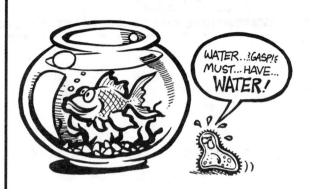

Explain that some germs are like fish—they live in liquids. A liquid is something you can pour or something that will drip. Water is a liquid.

2. Ask children to name some liquids that could be found at home in the refrigerator. As children respond, take sample refrigerator items out of the bag.

   Tell children to notice the different colors and thicknesses of the liquids. Point out that different liquids are used for different things.

3. Explain to children that the liquids inside our bodies are called fluids. The body contains different kinds of fluids. Help children think of different body fluids.

   Use the **New Words** section to determine which words are appropriate for the children in your class. Make sure you have word cards for the words you want to discuss.

   As fluids are named, place word cards on the bulletin board or in the chalk trays. As necessary and appropriate, discuss the meaning of each word.

4. Explain that some germs live inside the body in body fluids. These germs die if they are taken out of the fluid, just as the fish dies when it is removed from water. If we don't share body fluids, we will not share the germs that live in the fluids.

**Note to teacher**: There are certainly ways to share inside germs. If an inside germ, in saliva for instance, is transferred in a wet kiss from one person to another, the germ will stay in the fluid and will be passed on. Certain inside germs are passed on through sexual contact and from mother to unborn child through the amniotic fluid. The emphasis for children should be that it is not easy to share inside germs, but it does happen.

## New Words

amniotic fluid, blood, digestive juices, liquids, lymph, milk, mucus, saliva, semen, spinal fluids, sweat, tears, urine, vaginal fluids

## Where It Fits

health, science

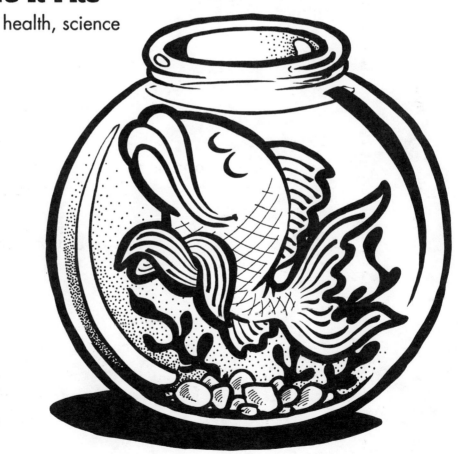

# Fish

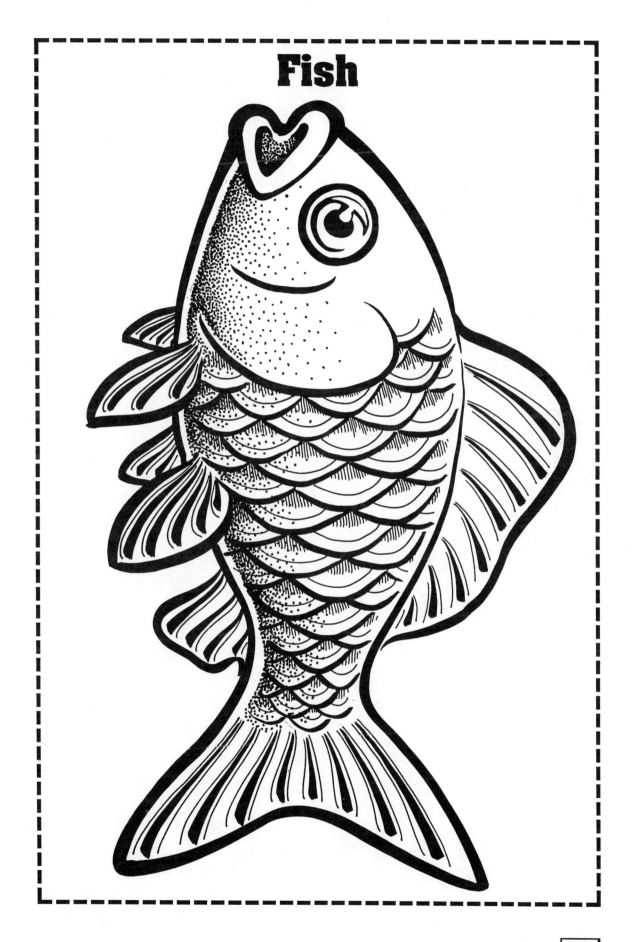

# 6 Keeping Germs Out

## Purpose

To help children understand how healthy skin helps keep germs out of the body.

## In a Nutshell

Children play a circle game that illustrates how skin keeps germs out. They talk about how to care for the skin.

## Get Ready, Get Set...

- Gather needed materials: 2 balloons, 2 clear containers (plastic peanut butter jars work well), clear baster (such as turkey baster).
- Fill 1 balloon with water; make several small holes in the other.
- Fill 1 container half-full of plain water. Fill the other half-full of dark colored water.
- Prepare word cards using *New Words*.

## Here We Go!

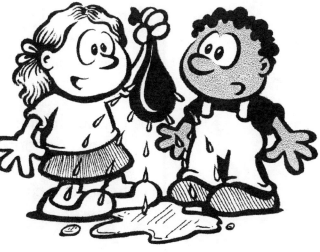

1. Ask children to name ways that our bodies keep germs out (skin is a barrier, tears kill germs, stomach fluids—"acids"—kill germs, etc.) Show children a balloon filled with water. Tell children the balloon

keeps the water inside the same way unbroken skin keeps what's inside our body safely in and what's outside safely out.

Show children a balloon with small holes in it. Show how water can get in or out of the holes. Tell children this is how broken skin allows germs (water) to enter. Ask children for examples of ways skin can be broken (cut, tear, puncture, scrape, picking at scabs).

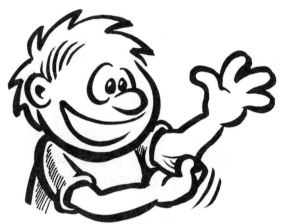

2. Tell children that the skin's ability to stretch helps keep it from tearing. This helps us keep germs outside our bodies. Have children gently pull the skin at their elbows to feel this stretching.

Ask children what would happen to the elbow skin if it were not stretchy. What other examples of skin's stretching can they think of?

Soft, stretchy skin is not as easy to tear as dry skin. Skin oils help keep our skin stretchy and soft. Tell children to look at their skin to see if it's dry.

Talk about things that make skin dry and chapped (weather, environmental conditions—heat, cold, humidity). What can we do to protect our skin? (Dress warmly in cold weather, put oil on dry skin, avoid cuts and scrapes, clean and cover breaks in the skin.)

3. Divide children into 2 groups. Have each group join hands and form a small circle. Tell children the circles represent the skin on 2 different bodies. Ask a child from each circle to step into the middle of the circle to represent germs.

# Germs Away!

## Activity Poster

ETR

turn page

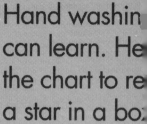

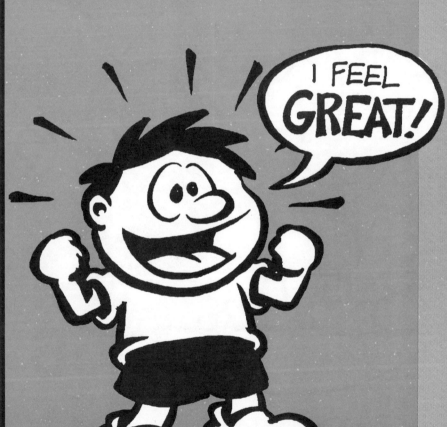

I FEEL GREAT!

Hand washin[g]
can learn. He[re]
the chart to re[...]
a star in a bo[x]

| Child's name |
| --- |
| After using t[he] |
| Before eating |
| When hand[s]<br>from play |
| (fill in your own) |

*Germs Away!* and its accompanying activity book, *Germ Smart,* are part of an exciting series of health act[...]

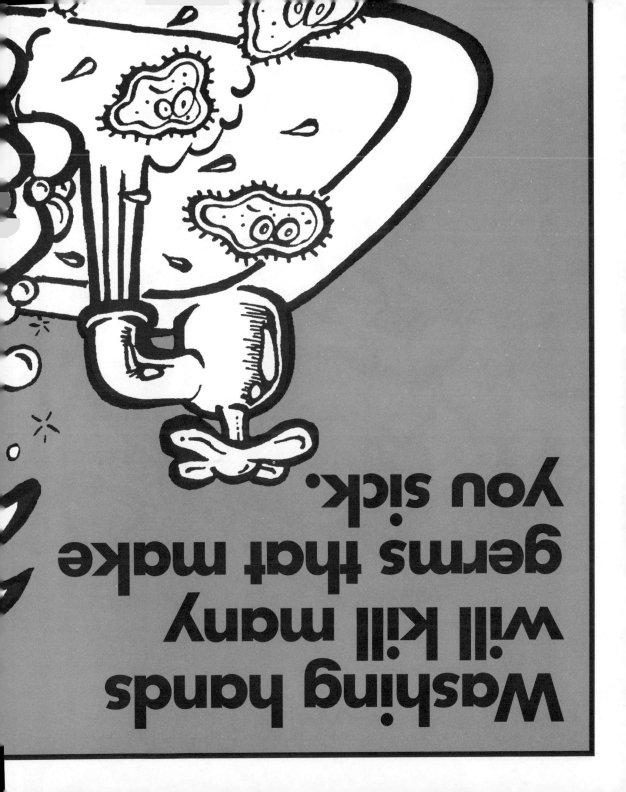

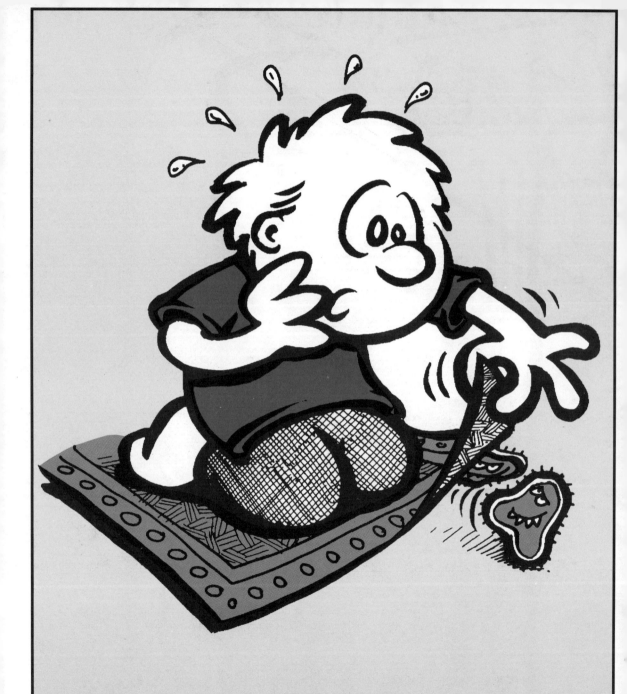

Germs are everywhere.

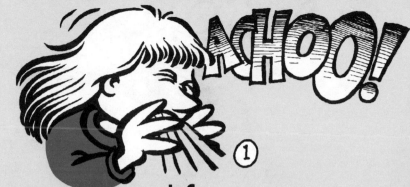

**ACHOO!**

Germs can spread from

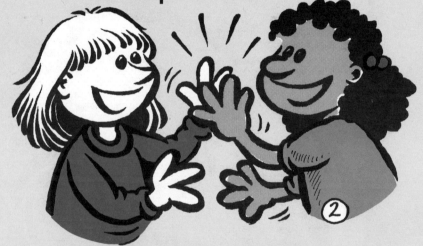

one person to another.

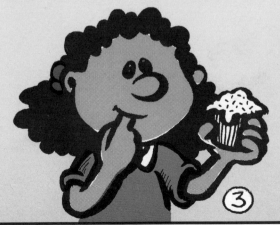

turn page

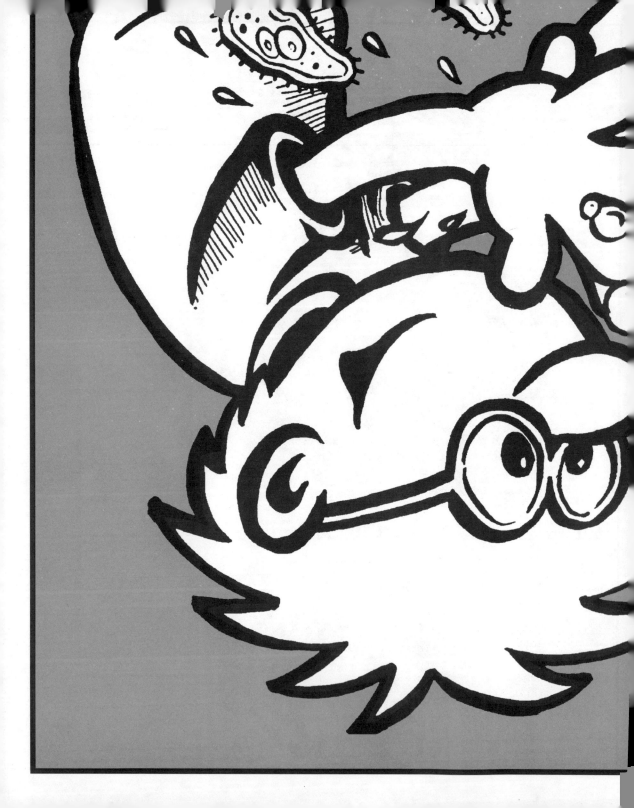

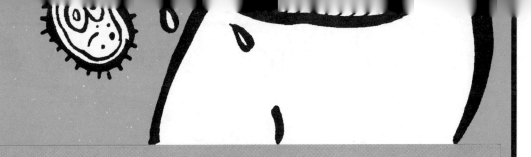

ne of the most important health behaviors children
d remind them to wash hands and stay healthy. Use
children when they wash their hands. Put a check or
en they remember.

| ⮞ ⮞ ⮞ | | | | |
|---|---|---|---|---|
| throom | | | | |
| | | | | |
| dirty | | | | |
| _____ | | | | |

ials by ETR Associates. For ordering information or to receive a free catalog, call 1-800-321-4407.

# They can get inside your body and make you sick.

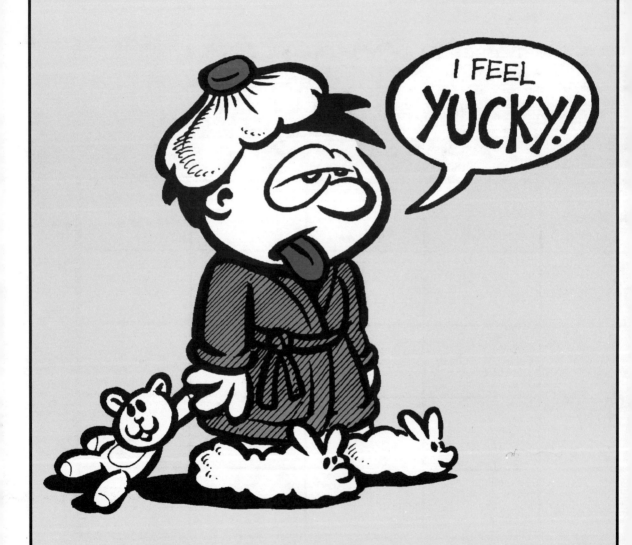

Now children can illustrate how the skin prevents these germs from spreading sickness to others. Tell the "germs" to gently attempt to move from their circle to the other. Tell the circles (skin) to keep the germs inside.

Now have children make a break in 1 circle to let their germ out. Point out that even though 1 germ got out of its circle, it can't get into the other circle. Germs

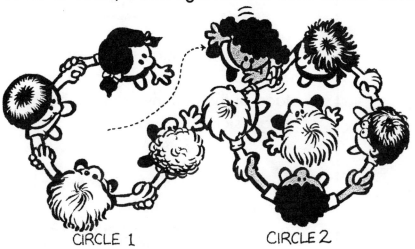

CIRCLE 1                    CIRCLE 2

cannot enter our bodies because unbroken skin keeps the germs out.

Have both circles illustrate broken skin. Allow the germs to pass freely from circle to circle (body to body). Demonstrate how cleaning and bandaging broken skin can help keep germs out.

4. Tell children that by learning what body fluids carry certain diseases (Concept 5), we can know what to do when we're around sick people.

Show children the clear containers, one half-filled with plain water to represent healthy body fluids and one half-filled with dark colored water to represent diseased body fluids. Show how these "bodies" can play together, sit together, bump together, share toys, etc., but the inside germs from one do not reach the other.

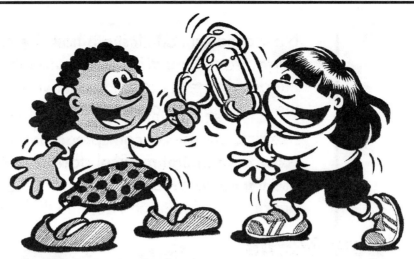

As long as the body fluid that contains the unwanted germ from an infected person does not get into the blood of the healthy person, the healthy person does not get sick.

5. Pour some clear water into the colored water to demonstrate transfusions. Point out that healthy blood can be shared under emergency conditions.

   Pour some colored water into the clear water to demonstrate that certain germs can be passed from person to person through transfusions. (This was the case, for example, with HIV, since it lives in blood.)

   Caution that certain activities that share blood have a high risk of spreading germs and disease. These activities should be carefully avoided. They include "blood brother or sister" games, making tattoos with shared needles and piercing ears with shared needles.

   Draw some of the colored water into

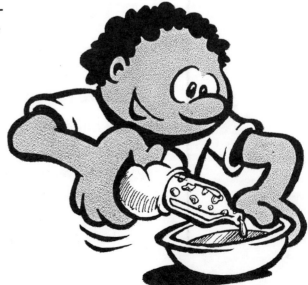

a clear baster. Empty the baster. Wipe off the colored droplets on the outside of the baster. Show children the droplets that remain inside.

Tell children that this is how blood can be left in used needles. The blood can spread deadly germs. Reassure children that medical doctors and nurses never use the same needle twice.

## New Words

chapped, needle, oil, stretch, transfusion

## Where It Fits

health, science

# 7 Fighting Germs

## Purpose

To help children understand how our bodies fight germs.

## In a Nutshell

Children see demonstrations of germ-fighting actions. They watch a puppet eat germs. They discuss good health habits.

## Get Ready, Get Set...

• Gather needed materials: clear container of white vinegar (without a label), another clear container, 1/4 cup baking soda, spoon or scoop, toothpicks, marbles or grapes.

• Fill a clear container half-full of dark-red colored water.

• Make a large-mouth puppet, such as a sock puppet, with a slit in the back of the mouth. Make a badge to attach to the puppet with Velcro. See the teacher page **Mac Puppet Directions.**

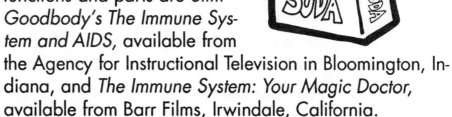

• Two excellent videos that describe the immune system's functions and parts are *Slim Goodbody's The Immune System and AIDS*, available from the Agency for Instructional Television in Bloomington, Indiana, and *The Immune System: Your Magic Doctor*, available from Barr Films, Irwindale, California.

• Prepare word cards using *New Words*.

# Here We Go!

1. Show children the container of white vinegar (a lid will conceal the smell) and the container of dark-red colored water. Explain that our blood contains white cells and red cells and a liquid called plasma. The red part (red water) carries food and fresh air to all parts of the body. The white cells (vinegar) fight germs that get past the skin and into the body.

   The white cells are part of the body's immune system. The immune system helps us fight germs and stay well.

2. Demonstrate how the white cells fight germs. Add a teaspoon of "pretend germs" (baking soda) to the white cells (vinegar). Compare the bubbling action that occurs to the fight between the white cells and the germs.

   Ask children what would happen if germs were put in with the red cells. (No action results.) Demonstrate this.

   Show children the vinegar (white cells) again. Add more germs (baking soda) until the bubbling stops. Explain that when germs enter our bodies the first time, the white cells fight very hard against the germs. Sometimes we don't know that a battle is being fought. Other times, we have a fever.

   Fever means your white cells are fighting with germs. After the battle, special white cells remember what that germ is like. If that germ tries to attack your body again, the white cells are ready to destroy it.

   Point out that the vinegar and baking-soda mixture looks cloudy. Tell children it has special white "memory cells" like those that remain in the body, waiting for the next germ attack.

Pour the vinegar and red water together. Remind children that although our blood looks red, it is really red and white cells mixed together along with plasma.

3. When our bodies fight infection, pus sometimes forms where the infection is. The sore place may also become swollen, reddish or feverish. Tell children that these are all signs that the body's immune system is fighting the germs.

Tell children there are several kinds of white cells in the immune system. The first cells to reach the invading germs are called macrophages (*mac' row fay jes*). These macrophages like to eat. They eat up the germs.

Use the puppet, Mac, to eat the germs. Use toothpicks for bacteria, and marbles or grapes for viruses. The puppet can appear to swallow the germs through the slit in the back of the mouth. Mac should call for help from other white cells and eat one or more germs.

After Mac eats the germs, place the Velcro badge on the puppet. Tell children the badge describes the germ invaders. Now the other types of white cells that come to help Mac (T-cells and B-cells) can learn from the badge exactly what they need to know about the germs.

4. Tell children that the immune system works every minute of every day to protect the body against germ invaders. When we are worried or upset, the im-

BADGE

mune system slows down. Our immune systems get stronger when we exercise, eat food that's good for us and get enough rest.

Talk with children about things that make them worried or upset (stress). Talk about ways to handle problems. Talk about how good health habits help our bodies stay strong. Explain the importance of exercise, rest, diet and cleanliness.

**Note to teacher:** Sometimes, in a few people, the immune system has been known to get "confused" and begin to attack its own body. That is what happens when a person has lupus, rheumatoid arthritis and possibly, multiple sclerosis.

## New Words

immune system, infection, macrophages, plasma, pus, red cells, swollen, white cells

## Where It Fits

health, science

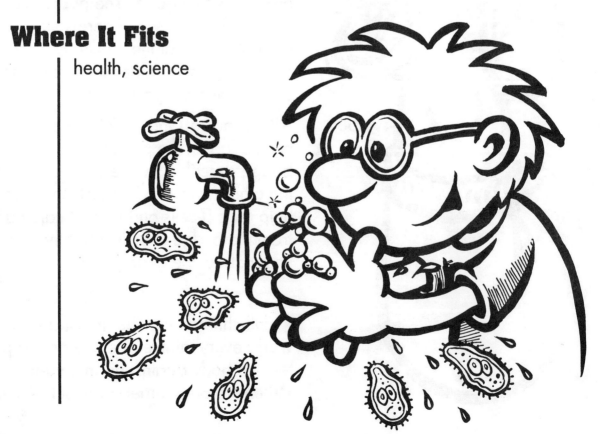

# Mac Puppet Directions

*Directions:* Obtain or make a puppet that has a large mouth. Put a slit in the back of the mouth that is not easily seen by children. Obtain a badge for Mac. Velcro will work on most puppet materials.

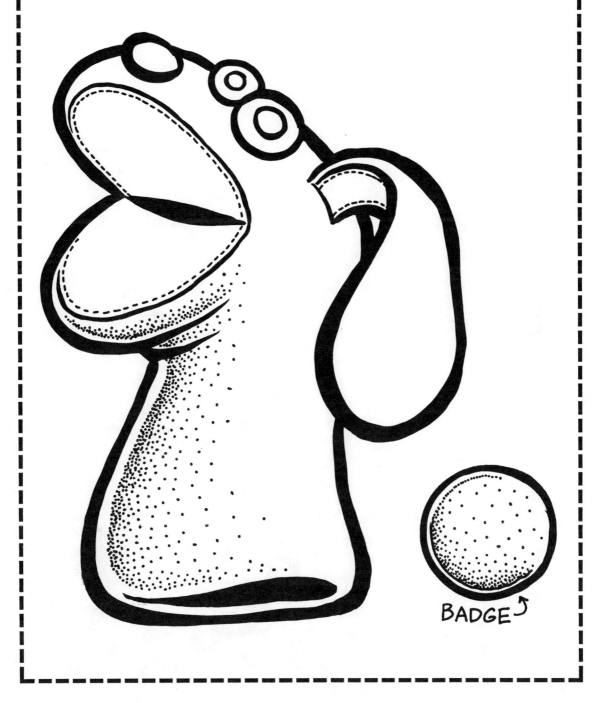

BADGE

# 8 Who's Sick?

## Purpose

To help children understand the relationship between behavior and health.

## In a Nutshell

Children see a continuum that illustrates degrees of health. They look at magazine pictures and guess who's infectious. They discuss signs and symptoms of disease.

## Get Ready, Get Set...

- Have magazine pictures of a variety of people, some who look well and some who are obviously ill.
- Review the **Story of Chad**.
- Prepare word cards using *New Words*.

## Here We Go!

1. Draw a 3-foot line on the chalkboard. Label one end HEALTHY and the other end VERY SICK. Draw a stick figure at the healthy end. Explain that this person is absolutely healthy—no diseases, no infections, no injuries, no cavities, not even a cough!

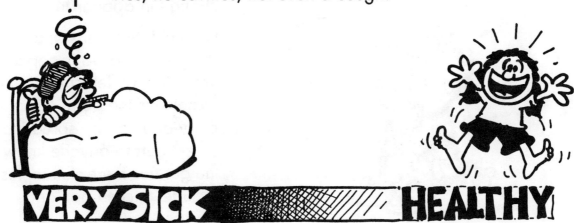

At the very sick end of the line, draw a figure lying in bed. Explain that this person is so sick that he or she is in a hospital or clinic for medical care.

Ask children to tell you where on this line to draw someone with a cold, with measles, a broken bone, 6 broken bones, 10 cavities, a sick heart, someone who's healthy and blind, healthy and pregnant. Draw and discuss each of these people. Point out that there are many different stages or degrees of health.

Ask children which of the people you have drawn might look healthy or well, even though they are not really in the best of health. Point out that we cannot always tell just by looking how someone really feels. Can we always tell when a person is sick? pregnant? has a sick heart? has cavities?

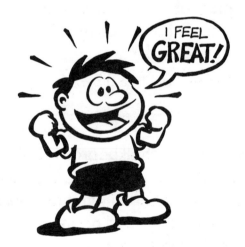

2. Explain that there are signs or symptoms that let us know that someone is sick or hurt. Ask children to name some common signs of someone who has a cold or measles or other sickness (pain, fever, tenderness, discoloration, loss of function, change in appearance, etc.).

Point out that signs and symptoms do not always appear immediately. Tell children that sometimes the germ enters the body and can be spread to others before anyone knows the germ is there. Examples include chicken pox and measles.

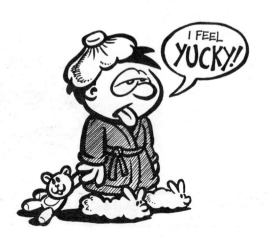

Show children magazine pictures of various people. Ask the children if they think each person could be infectious.

4. Draw another 3-foot line on the chalkboard. Label one end GREAT and the other end POOR. Use this to illustrate how a person's health can change from day to day because of choices they make.

Tell children the **Story of Chad**. Place an X on the line to indicate how Chad feels in the morning, at noon and in the evening of each day. Adapt or embellish each day's events to help children relate to Chad.

Conclude that our everyday actions affect how healthy we are and how well our bodies can fight off germs. If we take good care of our bodies, our immune systems will be able to take good care of us.

5. Review good health habits (rest, relaxation, foods that are good for us, cover coughs and sneezes, exercise or active play, cleanliness, do not share eating utensils). Talk with children about health helpers who can help us learn more about taking good care of our bodies. Health helpers include parents, doctor, nurse, teacher, other trusted adults.

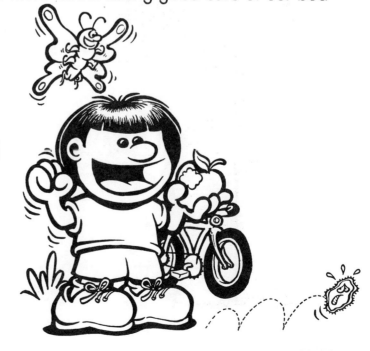

6. Tell children that germs are everywhere. We

can't always tell by looking who is sick and spreading germs. But we can act in ways that will help our bodies stay strong and fight germs.

## New Words

cavity, chicken pox, health helpers, infection, measles, pregnant

## Where It Fits

health, science

# The Story of Chad

Page 1

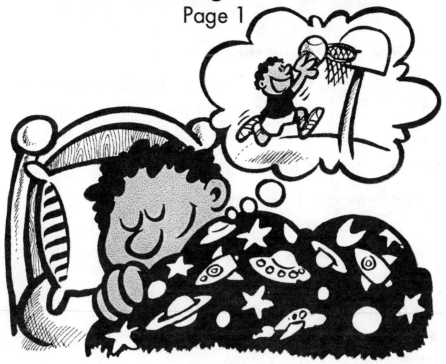

Thursday morning, Chad wakes up feeling wonderful. His cold is gone now. He can smell breakfast cooking. He feels rested and ready to go!

First he takes a shower. Then he brushes his teeth, eats a good breakfast and heads for school. At school, he works hard, exercises in gym class and plays ball during recess.

*Place an X on the line to show how Chad's decisions influence his health. (He is at GREAT.)*

Thursday afternoon, Chad skips lunch, snacks on candy and reads a book.

*Place an X on the line and discuss.*

Thursday evening, Chad skips dinner, goes to bed late and forgets to wash his hands after using the bathroom.

# The Story of Chad

*Place an X on the line and discuss.*

Friday morning, Chad wakes up tired, eats a good breakfast, but forgets to brush his teeth. He goes to school.

*Place an X on the line and discuss.*

Friday afternoon, Chad takes a nap after school, plays basketball, eats a good, healthy snack. He brushes his teeth after his snack and washes his hands before dinner.

*Place an X on the line and discuss.*

Friday night Chad takes a bath, brushes his teeth, relaxes and gets to bed on time.

*Place an X on the line and discuss.*

# 9 Tender Loving Care

## Purpose

To help children understand that there are many ways to show caring and concern to sick people.

## In a Nutshell

Children illustrate ways to show caring and concern for ill people. Children plot the location of community resources for a neighborhood map.

## Get Ready, Get Set...

- Prepare a simple neighborhood map of your community and copy one for each child. See the **Neighborhood Map Example.**
- Know the location of local public health agencies and other health care providers.
- Prepare word cards using *New Words.*

## Materials for Children

- ★ paper
- ★ pencil, crayons or markers
- ★ neighborhood map for each child

# Here We Go!

1. Ask children to think of times they have been sick. What did friends or family members do that made them feel better? Have children draw pictures of these helpful deeds.

2. Talk about what happens when someone is sick. Ask the following questions: Is the person who is sick the only one to suffer? How do people feel when someone they love is very sick? How are people affected by the illness of someone they love?

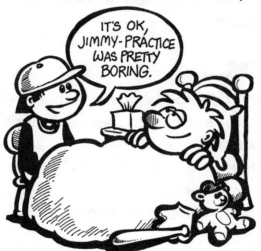

Talk to children about how important it is to show care and concern for people who are sick. Talk about showing care and concern to friends and family who are affected by a person's illness. Tell children that our illness can affect many others, so it is important that we keep ourselves well.

Help children identify ways that they can take better care of themselves. Discuss ways children can show the people who take care of them that they are ready, willing and able to take care of themselves.

3. Ask children the following questions: What if you came to school today and heard that a friend was sick? What would you need to know about the sickness before you could decide on a way to help? How can we learn about sickness?

4. Distribute the neighborhood maps. Help children plot the locations of the library and local health helpers.

## New Words

caring, concern

## Where It Fits

art, health, social studies

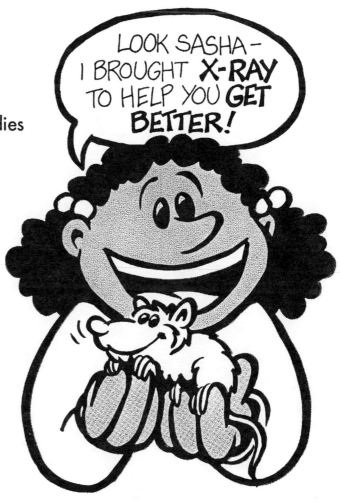

# Neighborhood Map Example

*Directions:* Make a simple map of your community. The following is provided as an example. Plot the location of the community resources with children in class.

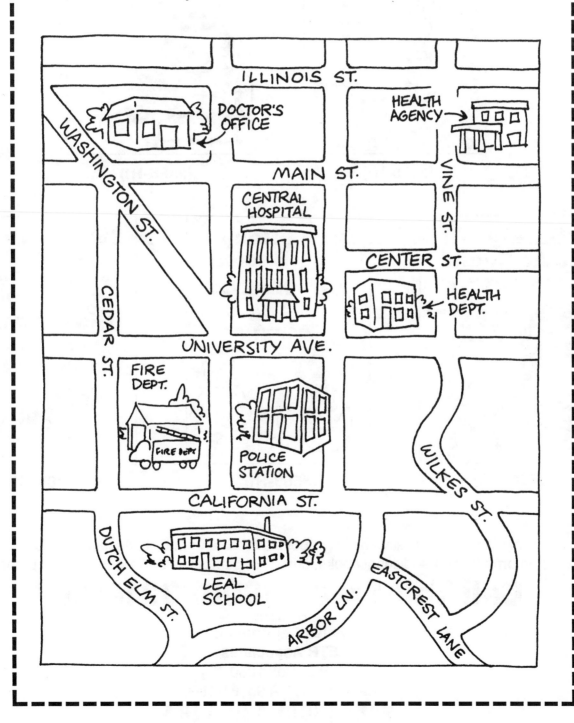

# More Hands-On Health Activity Books!

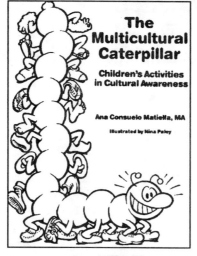

(#585-H1)

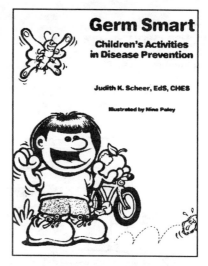

(#586-H1)

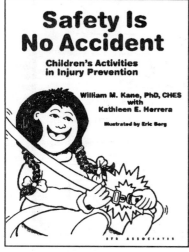

(#561-H1)

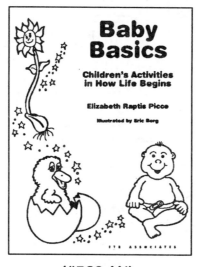

(#563-H1)

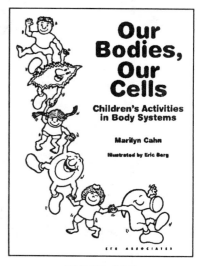

(#565-H1)

These are just a few of the creative activity books available from ETR Associates.  Don't miss out!
Call today for information on additional books, curricula, pamphlets and videos for the primary grades.

## Call Toll-Free 1 (800) 321-4407

or contact:
**Sales Department**
**ETR Associates**
P.O. Box 1830
Santa Cruz, CA 95061-1830
**FAX: (408) 438-4284**